Pescatarian Cookbook

Easy and Delicious Fish, Seafood and Vegetarian Recipes for a Healthy and Balanced Diet

Jacob Aiello

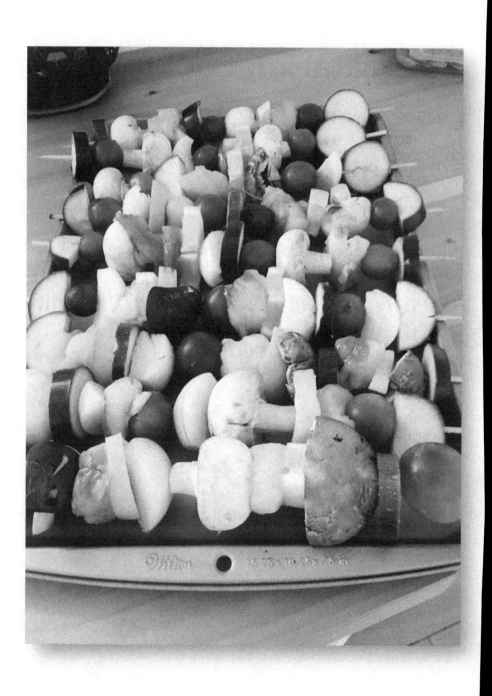

Table of Contents

by reading this document, the reader agrees that under no circumstances is the author responsible for any losses, direct or indirect, which are incurred as a result of the use of information contained within this document, including, but not limited to, — errors, omissions, or inaccuracies.

Fried Catfish

Servings: 4

Total Time: 60 Minutes

Calories: 208

Fat: 9 g

Protein: 17 g

Carbs: 8 g

Fiber: 0.6 g

Ingredients and Quantity

- 4 catfish fillets
- 1/4 cup seasoned fish fry (I used Louisiana)
- 1 tbsp. olive oil
- 1 tbsp. parsley, chopped, optional

Direction

1. Preheat air fryer to 400F.
2. Rinse the catfish and pat dry.
3. Pour the fish fry seasoning in a large Ziploc bag.
4. Add the catfish to the bag, one at a time. Seal the bag and shake. Ensure the entire filet is coated with seasoning.
5. Spray olive oil on the top of each filet.
6. Place the filet in the air fryer basket (due to the size of my fillets, I cooked each one at a time). Close and cook for 10 minutes.
7. Flip the fish. Cook for an additional 10 minutes.
8. Flip the fish. Cook for an additional 2-3 minutes or until desired crispness.
9. 10.Top with parsley. Serve and enjoy!

Lemony Vegan Salmon

Servings: 4

Total Time: 35 Minutes

Calories: 290

Fat: 16 g

Protein: 33 g

Carbs: 4 g

Fiber: 1 g

Ingredients and Quantity

- 2 tbsp. butter, melted
- 2 tbsp. green onions, sliced thinly
- 3/4 cup breadcrumbs, white, fresh
- 1/4 tsp. thyme leaves, dried
- 1 1/4 pounds salmon fillet, 1 piece
- 1/4 tsp. salt
- 1/4 cup vegan cheese, grated
- 2 tsp. lemon peel, grated

Direction

1. Preheat the air fryer at 350 degrees Fahrenheit.
2. Mist cooking spray onto a baking pan (shallow). Fill with pat-dried salmon.
3. Brush salmon with butter (1 tablespoon) before sprinkling with salt.
4. Combine the breadcrumbs with onions, thyme, lemon peel, cheese, and remaining butter (1 tablespoon).
5. Cover salmon with the breadcrumb mixture. Air-fry for fifteen totwenty-five minutes. Serve and enjoy!

Salmon Omelet

Servings: 2

Total Time: 18 Minutes

Calories: 193

Fat: 12.2 g

Protein: 19 g

Carbs: 1.3 g

Fiber: 0.1 g

Ingredients and Quantity

- 3 oz. smoked salmon, chopped
- 12 tbsp. apple sauce
- 1 tsp. scallions
- 1 pinch salt
- 1/4 tsp. ground black pepper
- 1/4 tsp. chili flakes
- 1/2 tsp. almond butter
- 2 tbsp. cream

Direction

1. Pour the apple sauce in a bowl.
2. Add the scallions and salt.
3. After this, sprinkle the apple sauce with the ground black pepper, chili flakes and cream.
4. Stir it carefully.
5. Preheat the air fryer to 360 F.
6. Toss the butter in the air fryer basket and melt it.
7. After this, pour the apple sauce mixture into the melted almond butter.
8. Add the chopped smoked salmon.
9. Cook the omelet for 8 minutes.
10. Transfer the cooked omelet onto the serving plates.
11. Serve and enjoy!

Golden Cod Fish Nuggets

Servings: 4

Total Time: 25 Minutes

Calories: 168

Fat: 7.7 g

Protein: 16.8 g

Carbs: 0.4 g

Fiber: 1.2 g

Ingredients and Quantity

- 4 cod fillets
- 2 tbsp. olive oil
- 4 tbsp. apple sauce
- 1 cup breadcrumbs
- A pinch salt

Direction

1. Preheat the Air Fryer to 390 F.
2. Place the breadcrumbs, olive oil, and salt in a food processor and process until evenly combined.
3. Pour the breadcrumb mixture into a bowl, the apple sauce into another bowl, and the flour into a third bowl.
4. Toss the cod fillets in the flour, then in the apple sauce, and then in the breadcrumb mixture.
5. Place them in the fryer basket, close and cook for 9 minutes.
6. At the 5-minute mark, quickly turn the chicken nuggets over.
7. Once golden brown, remove onto a serving plate and serve with vegetable fries. Enjoy!

Full Baked Trout en Papillote with Herbs

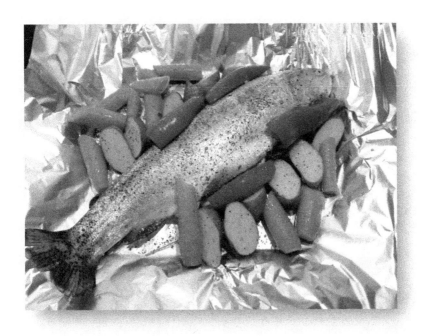

Servings: 2

Total Time: 30 Minutes

Calories: 243

Fat: 8.1 g

Protein: 15.6 g

Carbs: 2.9 g

Fiber: 0.4 g

Ingredients and Quantity

- 3/4 lb. whole trout, scaled and cleaned
- 1/4 bulb fennel, sliced
- 1/2 brown onion, sliced
- 3 tbsp. chopped parsley
- 3 tbsp. chopped dill
- 2 tbsp. olive oil
- 1 lemon, sliced
- Salt and pepper, to taste

Direction

1. In a bowl, add the onion, parsley, dill, fennel, and garlic. Mix and drizzle the olive oil over.
2. Preheat the Air Fryer to 350 F.
3. Open the cavity of the fish and fill with the fennel mixture.
4. Wrap the fish completely in parchment paper and then in foil.
5. Place the fish in the fryer basket and cook for 10 minutes.
6. Remove the paper and foil, and top with lemon slices.
7. Serve with a side of cooked mushrooms. Enjoy!

Breaded Scallops

Servings: 6

Total Time: 5 Minutes

Calories: 280

Fat: 32 g

Protein: 2.8 g

Carbs: 3.2 g

Fiber: 0.5 g

Ingredients and Quantity

- 12 fresh scallops
- 3 tbsp. almond flour
- 4 salt and black pepper
- 3 tbsp. apple sauce
- 1 cup breadcrumbs

Direction

1. Coat the scallops with flour.
2. Dip into the apple sauce, then into the breadcrumbs.
3. Spray them with olive oil and arrange them in the air fryer.
4. Cook for 6 minutes at 360 F, turning once halfway through cooking. Serve and enjoy!

Hot Salmon and Broccoli

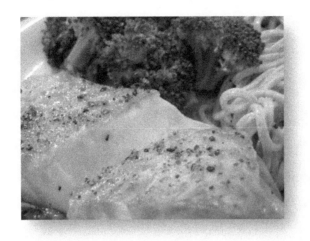

Servings: 2

Total Time: 25 Minutes

Calories: 368

Fat: 32 g

Protein: 4 g

Carbs: 5.8 g

Fiber: 3 g

Ingredients and Quantity

- 2 salmon fillets
- 1 tsp. olive oil
- Juice of 1 lime
- 1 tsp. chili flakes
- Salt and black pepper
- 1 head broccoli, cut into florets
- 1 tsp. olive oil
- 1 tbsp. soy sauce

Direction

1. In a bowl, add oil, lime juice, flakes, salt, and black pepper; rub the mixture onto fillets.
2. Lay the florets into your air fryer and drizzle with oil.
3. Arrange the fillets around or on top and cook at 340 F for 10 minutes.
4. Drizzle the florets with soy sauce to serve!

Soy Sauce Glazed Cod

Servings: 1

Total Time: 15 Minutes

Calories: 149

Fat: 5.8 g

Protein: 21 g

Carbs: 2.9 g

Fiber: 4 g

Ingredients and Quantity

- 1 cod fillet
- 1 tsp. olive oil
- A pinch sea salt
- A pinch pepper
- 1 tbsp. soy sauce
- Dash sesame oil
- 1/4 tsp. ginger powder
- 1/4 tsp. maple syrup

Direction

1. Preheat the Air fryer to 370 degrees.
2. Combine the olive oil, salt and pepper, and brush that mixture over the cod.
3. Place the cod onto an aluminum sheet and into the air fryer; cook for 6 minutes.
4. Meanwhile, combine the soy sauce, ginger, maple syrup, and sesame oil.
5. Brush the glaze over the cod.
6. Flip the fillet over and cook for 3 more minutes. Serve and enjoy!

County Baked Crab Cakes

Servings: 1

Total Time: 20 Minutes

Calories: 126

Fat: 5 g

Protein: 16 g

Carbs: 1.6 g

Fiber: 2 g

Ingredients and Quantity

- 1/2 pound jumbo crab
- Lemon juice, to taste
- 2 tbsp. parsley, chopped
- Old bay seasoning, as needed
- 1 tbsp. basil, chopped
- 3 tbsp. vegan mayo
- 1/4 tsp. Dijon mustard
- Zest of 1/2 lemo
- 1/4 cup panko breadcrumbs

Direction

1. Preheat your Fryer to 400 F, and in a bowl, mix mayo, lemon zest, old bay seasoning, mustard, and oil.
2. Blend crab meat in food processor and season with salt.
3. Transfer to the mixing bowl and combine well.
4. Form cakes using the mixture and dredge the mixture into breadcrumbs.
5. Place the cakes in your air fryer's basket and cook for 15 minutes.
6. Serve garnished with parsley and lemon juice. Enjoy!

Air Fried Salmon

Servings: 2

Total Time: 10 Minutes

Calories: 288

Fat: 19 g

Protein: 28 g

Carbs: 2 g

Fiber: 3 g

Ingredients and Quantity

- 2 wild caught salmon fillets with comparable thickness (about 1 1/12 inches thick)
- 2 tsp. avocado oil or olive oil
- 2 tsp. paprika
- Salt and coarse black pepper, to taste
- Lemon wedges

Direction

1. Remove any bones from your salmon (if necessary) and let fish sit on the counter for an hour.
2. Rub each fillet with olive oil and season with paprika, salt, and pepper.
3. Place fillets in the basket of the air fryer.
4. Set air fryer at 390 degrees for 7 minutes for 1½-inch fillets.
5. When timer goes off, open basket and check fillets with a fork to make sure they are done to your desired cook. Enjoy!

Air Fried Dragon Shrimp

Servings: 4

Total Time: 25 Minutes

Calories: 221

Fat: 13 g

Protein: 23 g

Carbs: 1 g

Fiber: 1.1 g

Ingredients and Quantity

- 1 pound raw shrimp, peeled and deveined 1/2 cup soy sauce
- 6 tbsp. apple sauce
- 2 tbsp. olive oil
- 1 cup yellow onion, diced
- 1/4 cup flour
- 1/2 tsp. red pepper, ground
- 1/2 tsp. ginger, grounded

Direction

1. Preheat your air fryer to 350 F.
2. Add all the ingredients except for the shrimp to make the batter.
3. Set it aside for 10 minutes.
4. Dip each shrimp into the batter to coat all sided.
5. Place them on the air fryer basket.
6. Cook for 10 minutes. Serve and enjoy!

Cheesy Haddock

Servings: 4

Total Time: 23 Minutes

Calories: 321

Fat: 15.7 g

Protein: 27.7 g

Carbs: 17 g

Ingredients and Quantity

- 4 haddock fillets
- 3/4 cup coconut milk
- 2 tsp. salt
- 3/4 cup bread crumbs
- 1/4 cup grated vegan cheese
- 1/4 tsp. ground dried thyme
- 1/4 cup almond butter, melted

Direction

1. Place in the ceramic pot the Foodi Cook and Crisp reversible rack.
2. Dip the haddock fillets in coconut milk then season with salt. Set aside.
3. In a mixing bowl, combine the bread crumbs, vegan cheese, and ground thyme.
4. Dredge the fillets in the bread crumbs mixture.
5. Place the fish on the reversible rack.
6. Brush withalmond butter on all sides.
7. Close the crisping lid and press the Bake/Roast button before pressing the Start button.
8. Adjust the cooking time to 20 minutes. Serve and enjoy!

Foil Baked Salmon

Servings: 2

Total Time: 23 Minutes

Calories: 619

Fat: 51.3 g

Protein: 36.3 g

Carbs: 2.9 g

Ingredients and Quantity

- 2 salmon fillets
- 2 garlic cloves, minced
- 6 tbsp. olive oil
- 1 tsp. dried basil
- 1 tsp. salt
- 1 tsp. ground black pepper
- 1 tbsp. lemon juice
- 1 tbsp. fresh parsley, chopped

Direction

1. Place in the ceramic pot the Foodi Cook and Crisp reversible rack.
2. On a large foil, place the salmon fillets and season with the rest of the ingredients.
3. Do not fold the aluminum foil.
4. Place the foil - fish and all - on the reversible tray.
5. Close the crisping lid and press the Bake/Roast button before pressing the START button.
6. Adjust the cooking time to 20 minutes or until the fish is flaky. Serve and enjoy!

Pasta with Capers and Tuna

Servings: 4

Total Time: 25 Minutes

Ingredients and Quantity

- 1 tbsp. olive oil
- 1 garlic clove
- 3 anchovies
- 2 cups tomato puree
- 1 1/2 tsp. salt
- 16 oz. (500 g) fusilli pasta
- Two 5 1/2 oz. (160 g) cans Tuna packed in olive oil
- water to cover
- 2 tbsp. capers

Direction

1. In the pre-heated Foodi Multicooker on "Sauté" mode, add the oil, garlic and anchovies.
2. Sauté until the anchovies begin to disintegrate and the garlic cloves are just starting to turn golden.

3. Add the tomato puree and salt and mix together.
4. Pour in the uncooked pasta, and the contents of one tuna can (5 oz.) mixing to coat the dry pasta evenly.
5. Flatten the pasta in an even layer and pour in just enough water to cover.
6. Lock the lid on the Foodi Multicooker and then cook for 3 minutes. To get 3-minutes cook time, press "Pressure" button and use the Time Adjustment button to adjust the cook time to 3 minutes.
7. When time is up, open the cooker by releasing the pressure.
8. Mix in the last 5 oz. of tuna.
9. Close crisping lid and select Broil, set time to 7 minutes.
10. 10.Sprinkle with capers before serving. Enjoy!

Tuna Bowls

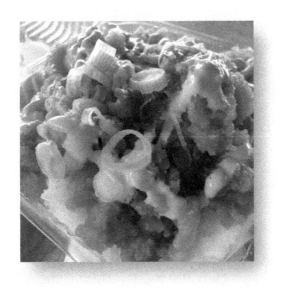

Servings: 4

Total Time: 13 Minutes

Calories: 202

Fat: 7 g

Protein: 6 g

Carbs: 12 g

Fiber: 7 g

Ingredients and Quantity

- 16 oz. canned tuna, drained and flaked
- 1 red onion, chopped
- A handful baby spinach
- 1 tbsp. lime juice
- 2 spring onions, chopped
- 3 tbsp. butter, melted

Direction

1. Set the Foodi on Sauté mode, add the butter, heat it up, add the onion, stir and cook for 2 minutes.
2. Add the rest of the ingredients, toss.
3. Put the pressure lid on and cook on High for 5-6 minutes.
4. Release the pressure fast for 5 minutes.
5. Divide everything into bowls and serve. Enjoy!

Ranch Fish Fillet

Servings: 4

Total Time: 30 Minutes

Calories: 425

Fat: 25.4 g

Protein: 18.8 g

Carbs: 30.4 g

Ingredients and Quantity

- 3/4 cup bread crumbs
- 1 packet dry ranch dressing mix
- 2 1/2 tbsp. vegetable oil
- 6 tbsp. apple sauce
- fish fillets

Direction

1. Combine the bread crumbs and ranch mix in a bowl.
2. Pour in the oil.

3. Dip each fish fillet into the apple sauce and cover with the crumb mixture.
4. Place in the Ninja Foodi basket and seal the lid.
5. Select air crisp function.
6. Cook at 360 degrees F for 12 minutes, flipping halfway through.
7. You can garnish with lemon wedges. Enjoy!

Paprika Salmon

Servings: 2

Total Time: 25 Minutes

Calories: 248

Fat: 11.9 g

Protein: 34.9 g

Carbs: 1.5 g

Ingredients and Quantity

- 2 salmon fillets
- 2 tsp. avocado oil
- 2 tsp. paprika
- Salt and pepper, to taste

Direction

1. Coat the salmon with oil.
2. Season with salt, pepper and paprika.
3. Place in the Ninja Foodi basket.

4. Select the air crisp function.

5. Seal the crisping lid.

6. Cook at 390 degrees for 7 minutes.

7. You can garnish with lemon slices. Enjoy!

Fish Sticks

Servings: 2

Total Time: 25 Minutes

Calories: 549

Fat: 15 g

Protein: 61 g

Carbs: 39.4 g

Ingredients and Quantity

- 1 lb. cod, sliced into strips
- 1/2 cup tapioca starch
- 2 eggs
- 1 tsp. dried dill
- Salt and pepper, to taste
- 1 cup almond flour
- 1 tsp. onion powder
- 1/2 tsp. mustard powder
- 2 tbsp. avocado oil

Direction

1. Pat the cod fillet strips dry using paper towel.
2. Place the tapioca starch in a bowl.
3. In another bowl, beat the eggs.
4. In a larger bowl, mix the dill, salt, pepper, almond flour, onion powder and mustard powder.
5. Dip each strip in the first, second and third bowls.
6. Coat the Ninja Foodi basket with the avocado oil.
7. Place the fish strips inside. Cook at 390 degrees F for 5 minutes.
8. You can serve with tartar sauce. Enjoy!

Fish Fillet with Pesto Sauce

Servings: 3

Total Time: 28 Minutes

Calories: 383

Fat: 22.6 g

Protein: 42.1 g

Carbs: 2.2 g

Ingredients and Quantity

- 3 white fish fillets
- 1 tbsp. olive oil
- Salt and pepper, to taste
- 2 cups fresh basil leaves
- 2 garlic cloves, crushed
- 2 tbsp. pine nuts
- tbsp. vegan cheese, grated
- cup olive oil

Direction

1. Coat the fish fillets with 1 tablespoon of olive oil.
2. Season with the salt and pepper.
3. Place in the Ninja Foodi basket.
4. Cook at 320 degrees for 8 minutes.
5. While waiting, mix the remaining ingredients in a food processor.
6. Pulse until smooth.
7. Spread the pesto sauce on both sides of the fish before serving.
8. You can garnish with chopped pine nuts. Enjoy!

Hot Crispy Prawns

Servings: 4

Total Time: 25 Minutes

Calories: 490

Fat: 27.8 g

Protein: 0.3 g

Carbs: 8.7 g

Ingredients and Quantity

- 1 tsp. chili flakes
- 1 tsp. chili powder
- Salt and pepper, to taste
- 12 king prawns
- 3 tbsp. vegan mayonnaise
- 1 tbsp. ketchup
- 1 tbsp. wine vinegar

Direction

1. Combine all the spices in a bowl.
2. Toss the prawns in the spice mixture.
3. Place the prawns in the Ninja Foodi basket.
4. Seal the crisping lid.
5. Choose air crisp function.
6. Cook at 360 degrees for 8 minutes.
7. While waiting, mix the vegan mayo, ketchup and vinegar.
8. Serve with the prawns. Enjoy!

Crispy Shrimp

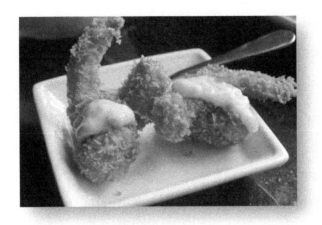

Servings: 4

Total Time: 30 Minutes

Calories: 229

Fat: 4.9 g

Protein: 30.7 g

Carbs: 13.8 g

Ingredients and Quantity

- 1 lb. shrimp, peeled and deveined
- 4 tbsp. apple sauce

- 1/2 cup bread crumbs
- 1/2 cup onion, diced
- 1 tsp. ginger1 tsp. garlic powder
- Salt and pepper, to taste

Direction

1. In one bowl, beat the two eggs.
2. In another bowl, put the rest of the ingredients.
3. Dip the shrimp first in the apple sauce and then in the spice mixture.
4. Place in the Ninja Foodi basket.
5. Seal the crisping lid.
6. Choose air crisp function.
7. Cook at 350 degrees for 10 minutes.
8. You can serve with chili sauce. Enjoy!

Cream of Zucchini Soup

Servings: 4

Total Time: 5 Hours 10 Minutes

Calories: 79

Fat: 10 g

Protein: 5 g

Carbs: 4.3 g

Ingredients and Quantity

- 1 tbsp. coconut cream
- 1/4 tbsp. pepper
- 1 tbsp. almond butter
- 1/2 cup chopped yellow onion
- 2 cups vegetable broth
- 4 cups chopped with peel green zucchini squash

Direction

1. Mix all the ingredients in your crock pot just leaving out the coconut cream.
2. Cook for about 5 hours on low or until zucchini is tender-soft.
3. Puree the soup in a blender.
4. Stir in the coconut cream then serve. Enjoy!

Low Carb Vegetable Soup

Servings: 6

Total Time: 8 Hours 10 Minutes

Calories: 125.2

Fat: 3.9 g

Protein: 11.9 g

Carbs: 11.6 g

Ingredients and Quantity

- 8 oz. fresh mushrooms, sliced
- 2 cans (14 oz.) vegetable broth
- 1 can diced tomatoes
- 1 green pepper, chopped
- 1 yellow onion, chopped
- 1 zucchini, thinly sliced
- 4 oz. turkey, sliced
- Vegan cheese, for topping
- 1 tsp. stevia

- 1 1/2 tbsp. basil leaves
- 1/2 tsp. salt

Direction

1. Put the broth, veggies, tomatoes, stevia, salt and basil in a slow cooker and mix thoroughly.
2. Top with the turkey slices then cook on low for 8 hours or high for 4 hours.
3. Pour into bowls and top with the cheese. Serve and enjoy!

Seafood Stew

Servings: 6

Total Time: 8 Hours 10 Minutes

Calories: 117.4

Fat: 5.8 g

Protein: 25.2 g

Carbs: 4.7 g

Ingredients and Quantity

- 2 tbsp. fresh parsley, chopped
- 1/2 tsp. salt
- 1 tsp. dried basil leaves
- 1/4 tsp. red pepper sauce
- 2 tbsp. olive oil
- 1 cup baby carrots, sliced
- 3 cups sliced quartered Roma tomatoes
- 1 tsp. Splenda
- 1/2 cup green bell pepper, chopped
- 1 cup water

- 1/2 tsp. fennel seed
- 1/2 lb. peeled and deveined shrimp
- 1 lb. cod cut into 1 inch slices
- 2 garlic cloves, finely chopped

Direction

1. Mix garlic and oil in a crockpot. Add tomatoes, carrots, fennel seed, bell pepper, clam juice and water then stir.
2. Cover and cook for 8 to 9 hours on low heat or until the vegetables are tender.
3. Around 20 minutes before serving, stir in the shrimp, cod, basil, splenda, pepper sauce and salt.
4. Cover and cook on high until the fish flakes with a fork.
5. Add in the parsley and stir. Serve and enjoy!

Tuna and White Beans Salad

Servings: 6

Total Time: 9 Hours 15 Minutes

Calories: 468

Fat: 15.5 g

Protein: 35.8 g

Carbs: 48.4 g

Ingredients and Quantity

- 4 tbsp. extra virgin olive oil
- 1 garlic clove, crushed and minced
- 1 lb. white beans, soaked overnight, rinsed and drained
- 6 cups water
- 14 oz. canned white tuna in water, drained and shredded
- 2 cups tomatoes, chopped
- 2 tsp. dried basil
- Salt and pepper, to taste
- 1 bunch Romaine lettuce, chopped

Direction

1. Add the olive oil to a skillet. Sauté the garlic for 1 minute.
2. Remove the garlic from the pan.
3. Cook the beans in the slow cooker on low for 3 hours.
4. Add the garlic-flavored olive oil.
5. Pour the water into the pot.
6. Cover and set it on high. Cook for 1 hour.
7. Reduce the temperature to low.
8. Cook for another 5 hours.
9. Add the tuna, tomatoes and basil. Mix well.
10. Arrange the lettuce in salad bowls.
11. Top with the tuna and beans mixture. Serve and enjoy!

Shrimp Creole

Servings: 6

Total Time: 4 Hours 15 Minutes

Calories: 346

Fat: 3.2 g

Protein: 39 g

Carbs: 38.9 g

Ingredients and Quantity

- 1 1/4 cups onion, chopped
- 1 garlic clove, crushed and minced
- 1 cup red bell pepper, chopped
- 1 1/2 cups celery, diced
- 1 tsp. salt
- 1/4 tsp. pepper
- 6 drops Tabasco
- 1/2 tsp. Creole seasoning
- 8 oz. canned tomato sauce
- 28 oz. canned whole tomatoes, crushed

- 2 lb. shrimp, deveined and shell removed
- 1 cup white rice, cooked

Direction

1. Add all the ingredients to the slow cooker, except for the shrimp.
2. Cook on High for 4 hours.
3. In the last 30 minutes of your cooking, add the shrimp.
4. Put hot, cooked rice in a bowl.
5. Top with the shrimp. Serve and enjoy!

Salmon and Scalloped Potatoes

Servings: 9

Total Time: 9 Hours 15 Minutes

Calories: 174

Fat: 4.2 g

Protein: 12.4 g

Carbs: 22.2 g

Ingredients and Quantity

- Cooking spray
- 3 tbsp. flour
- Salt and pepper, to taste
- 16 oz. salmon, drained and shredded into flakes
- 5 potatoes, sliced
- 1/2 cup onion, chopped
- 1/4 cup water
- 10 oz. cream of mushroom soup
- Pinch of nutmeg

Direction

1. Grease your slow cooker with cooking spray.
2. Sprinkle with a little bit of flour.
3. Sprinkle with salt and pepper.
4. Arrange a layer of half of the salmon flakes, half of the potatoes, and half of the chopped onions.
5. Make another set of layers.
6. In a bowl, mix the water and soup.
7. Pour into the slow cooker. Add the nutmeg.
8. Cover the pot. Cook on low for 9 hours. Serve and enjoy!

Tilapia in Lemon Pepper Sauce

Servings: 4

Total Time: 2 Hours 30 Minutes

Calories: 172

Fat: 7.2 g

Protein: 23.6 g

Carbs: 4.7 g

Ingredients and Quantity

- 4 fillets tilapia
- 16 spears asparagus
- 8 tbsp. freshly squeezed lemon juice
- 8 tbsp. pepper
- 2 tbsp. almond butter

Direction

1. Cut a foil that's large enough to wrap around the tilapia fillet.
2. Put each tilapia fillet into a foil.
3. Place 4 spears of asparagus on each tilapia.
4. Sprinkle each fillet with ¼ teaspoon pepper.
5. Sprinkle 2 tablespoons lemon juice onto each fillet.
6. Add ½ tablespoon butter on each fillet.
7. Wrap the fillet with the foil.
8. Place wrapped tilapia in the slow cooker.
9. Put on the lid and cook on High for 2 hours. Serve and enjoy!

Shrimp Scampi

Servings: 4

Total Time: 2 Hours 10 Minutes

Calories: 180

Fat: 7.1 g

Protein: 21.5 g

Carbs: 3.5 g

Ingredients and Quantity

- 1/2 cup white wine
- 1/4 cup reduced sodium chicken stock
- 2 tbsp. freshly squeezed lemon juice
- 2 tsp. parsley, minced
- 2 tsp. garlic, chopped2 tbsp. olive oil
- 1 lb. large shrimp (about 16 to 20 pieces)

Direction

1. Mix all the ingredients in a large bowl.
2. Transfer to the slow cooker.
3. Cook on low for 2 hours.
4. Serve in bowls. Enjoy!

VEGETARIAN RECIPES

The vegetarian recipes in this cookbook were inspired by the Mediterranean lifestyle, which helps you cook delicious meals with healthy, locally available ingredients that you can buy or even grow in your backyard. Some of the commonly used ingredients in these vegetarian recipes include: extra virgin olive oil, fresh vegetables, protein-rich legumes, nuts, seeds, healthy cheeses, aromatic, super food herbs and spices.

All Mediterranean vegetarian dishes are generally prepared slowly in an all-in-one pot and are very rarely fried. Another benefit of vegetarian meal is that they usually have low WW food point scores, most of the dishes even have zero point score. This helps you achieve your weight loss set target within the possible shortest period of time. Not only that, you will also enjoy delicious meals while still meeting your healthy lifestyle and weight loss target. The meals in this cookbook will keep you free from digestion problems, excess weight gain, diabetes and also keep you free from heart diseases.

You will find in this cookbook, delicious vegetarian soups and salads recipes that can serve as main meal, side dish or even use it to garnish your seafood dishes.

Air Fried Zucchini Chips

Servings: 3

Total Time: 20 Minutes

Calories: 187

Fat: 6.6 g

Protein: 10.8 g

Carbs: 21.1 g

Ingredients and Quantity

- 1 cup panko bread crumbs
- 3/4 grated vegan cheese
- 1 medium zucchini, sliced thinly
- 3 tbsp. apple sauce

Direction

1. Place the Ninja Foodi Cook and Crisp basket in the ceramic pot.
2. Mix the panko bread crumbs and parmesan cheese. Set aside.
3. Dip the zucchini in apple sauce before dredging in the panko mixture.
4. Place the dredged zucchini in the basket.
5. Close the crisping lid and press the Air Crisp button before pressing the START button.
6. Adjust the cooking time to 15 minutes. Serve and enjoy!

Crispy Cauliflower Bites

Servings: 4

Total Time: 12 Minutes

Calories: 130

Fat: 7 g

Protein: 4.3 g

Carbs: 12.4 g

Ingredients and Quantity

- 3 garlic cloves, minced
- 1 tbsp. olive oil
- 1/2 tsp. salt
- 1/2 tsp. smoked paprika
- 4 cups cauliflower florets

Direction

1. Place in the ceramic pot the Foodi Cook and Crisp basket.
2. Place all ingredients in a bowl and toss to combine.
3. Place the seasoned cauliflower florets in the basket.

4. Close the crisping lid and press the Air Crisp button before pressing the START button.
5. Adjust the cooking time to 10 minutes.
6. Give the basket a shake while cooking for even cooking. Serve and enjoy!

Baked Bananas

Servings: 4

Total Time: 12 Minutes

Calories: 183

Fat: 0.9 g

Protein: 1.4 g

Carbs: 42.2 g

Ingredients and Quantity

- 4 firm bananas, peeled and halved
- 1/4 cup maple syrup
- 1 tbsp. ground cinnamon
- 1 piece fresh ginger, grated
- 1 1/2 tsp. nutmeg

Direction

1. Place in the ceramic pot the Foodi Cook and Crisp reversible rack.

2. In a bowl, season the bananas with maple syrup, ground cinnamon, ginger, and nutmeg.

3. Place the bananas on the rack.

4. Close the crisping lid and press the Bake/Roast button before pressing the START button.

5. Adjust the cooking time to 10 minutes. Serve and enjoy!

Spicy Roasted Broccoli

Servings: 2

Total Time: 23 Minutes

Calories: 76

Fat: 3.9 g

Protein: 2.1 g

Carbs: 8 g

Ingredients and Quantity

- 2 cups broccoli florets
- 1 yellow bell pepper, sliced
- 1 tsp. garlic powder
- 1 tbsp. steak seasoning
- 2 tsp. chili powder
- 1 tbsp. extra virgin olive oil
- Salt and pepper, to taste

Direction

1. Place in the ceramic pot the Foodi Cook and Crisp basket insert.
2. Toss all ingredients in a mixing bowl.
3.
4. Place the vegetables in the basket.
5. Close the crisping lid and press the Bake/Roast button before pressing the START button.
6. Adjust the cooking time to 20 minutes.
7. Give the basket a shake to roast the veggies evenly. Serve and enjoy!

Quinoa and Potato Salad

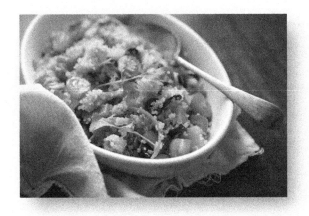

Servings: 6

Total Time: 25 Minutes

Ingredients and Quantity

- 1/4 cup white balsamic vinegar
- 1 tbsp. Dijon mustard
- 1 tsp. sweet paprika
- 1/2 tsp. ground black pepper
- 1/4 tsp. celery seeds
- 1/4 tsp. salt
- 1/4 cup olive oil
- 1 1/2 pounds tiny white potatoes, halved

- 1 cup blond (white) quinoa
- 1 medium shallot, minced
- 2 medium celery stalks, thinly sliced
- 1 large dill pickle, diced

Direction

1. Whisk the vinegar, mustard, paprika, pepper, celery seeds and salt in a large serving bowl until smooth.
2. Whisk in the olive oil in a thin, steady stream until the dressing is fairly creamy.
3. Place the potatoes and quinoa in the Ninja Foodi Multicooker; add enough cold tap water so that the ingredients are submerged by 3 inches (some of the quinoa may float).
4. Lock the lid on the Ninja Foodi Multicooker and then cook for 10 minutes. To get 10-minutes cook time, press "Pressure" button and use the Time Adjustment button to adjust the cook time to 10 minutes.
5. Use the quick-release method to bring the pot's pressure back to normal.
6. Unlock and open the pot. Close the crisping lid.
7. Select BROIL, and set the time to 5 minutes. Select START/STOP to begin.
8. Cook until top has browned.

9. Drain the contents of the pot into a colander lined with paper towels or into a fine-mesh sieve in the sink. Do not rinse.

10. Transfer the potatoes and quinoa to the large bowl with the dressing.

11. Add the shallot, celery, and pickle; toss gently and set aside for a minute or two to warm up the vegetables. Serve and enjoy!

Buttery Carrots with Pancetta

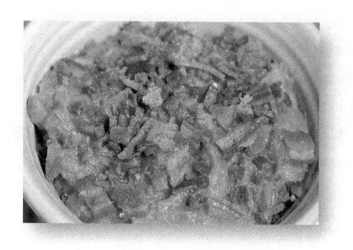

Servings: 5

Total Time: 20 Minutes

Ingredients and Quantity

- 4 oz. pancetta, diced
- 1 medium leek, white and pale green parts only, sliced lengthwise, washed and thinly sliced
- 1/4 cup moderately sweet white wine (I used dry Riesling)
- 1 pound baby carrots
- 1/2 tsp. ground black pepper
- 2 tbsp. almond butter, cut into small bits

Direction

1. Put the pancetta in the Ninja Foodi turned to the Air Crisp function.
2. Use time adjustment button to set cooking time to 5 minutes.
3. Add the leeks; cook, often stirring, until softened.
4. Pour in the wine and scrape up any browned bits at the bottom of the pot as it comes to a simmer.
5. Add the carrots and pepper; stir well.
6. Scrape and pour the contents of the Ninja Foodi Multicooker into a 1-quart, round, high-sided soufflé or baking dish. Dot with the bits of butter.
7. Lay a piece of parchment paper on top of the dish, then a piece of aluminum foil.
8. Seal the foil tightly over the baking dish.
9. Set the Ninja Foodi Multicooker rack inside, and pour in 2 cups water.
10. Use aluminum foil to build a sling for the baking dish; lower the baking dish into the cooker.
11. Lock the lid on the Ninja Foodi Multicooker and then cook for 7 minutes. To get 7-minutes cook time, press "Pressure" button and use the Time Adjustment button to adjust the cook time to 7 minutes.
12. Use the quick-release method to return the pot's pressure to normal.

13. Close the crisping lid. Select BROIL, and set the time to 5 minutes.
14. Select START/STOP to begin. Cook until top has browned.
15. Unlock and open the pot. Use the foil sling to lift the baking dish out of the cooker.
16. Uncover and stir well. Serve and enjoy!

Almond Butter Spaghetti Squash

Servings: 6

Total Time: 25 Minutes

Ingredients and Quantity

- One 3 1/2 pound spaghetti squash
- 6 tbsp. almond butter
- 2 tbsp. packed fresh sage leaves, minced
- 1/2 tsp. salt
- 1/2 tsp. ground black pepper
- 1/2 cup finely grated vegan cheese (about 1 oz.)

Direction

1. Put the squash with the cut side facing up in the cooker. Then add 1 cup water.
2. Lock the lid on the Ninja Foodi and then cook for 12 minutes.

3. Use the quick-release method to bring the pot's pressure back to normal.
4. Unlock and open the cooker. Transfer the squash halves to a cutting board; cool for 10 minutes.
5. Discard the liquid in the cooker.
6. Use a fork to scrape the spaghetti-like flesh off the skin and onto the cutting board; discard the skins.
7. Melt the butter in the electric cooker turned to its browning function.
8. Stir in the sage, salt, and pepper, then add all of the squash.
9. Stir and toss over the heat until well combined and heated through about 2 minutes.
10. Add the cheese, toss well. Close the crisping lid.
11. Select BROIL, and set the time to 5 minutes.
12. Select START/STOP to begin.
13. Cook until top has browned. Serve and enjoy!

Rye Berry and Celery Root Salad

Servings: 6

Total Time: 45 Minutes

Ingredients and Quantity

- 3/4 cup rye berries
- 1 medium celeriac (celery root), peeled and shredded through the large holes of a box grater
- 2 tbsp. almond butter
- 2 tbsp. maple syrup
- 2 tbsp. apple cider vinegar
- 1/2 tsp. salt
- 1/2 tsp. ground black pepper

Direction

1. Place the rye berries in the Foodi; pour in enough cold tap water, so the grains are submerged by 2 inches.
2. Lock the lid on the Foodi and then cook for 40 minutes.

3. Pressure Release. Use the quick-release method to bring the pot's pressure back to normal.
4. Unlock and open the cooker. Stir in the shredded celeriac.
5. Cover the pot without locking it and set aside for 1 minute.
6. Drain the pot into a large colander set in the sink.
7. Wipe out the cooker. Melt the butter in the Foodi; turned to it sauté function.
8. Add the maple syrup and cook for 1 minute, constantly stirring.
9. Add the drained rye berries and celeriac; cook, constantly stirring, for 1 minute.
10. 10.Stir in the vinegar, salt, and pepper to serve. Enjoy!

Crispy Tofu

Servings: 4

Total Time: 60 Minutes

Calories: 137

Fat: 3.4 g

Protein: 2.3 g

Carbs: 24 g

Ingredients and Quantity

- 1 tsp. seasoned rice vinegar
- 2 tbsp. low sodium soy sauce
- 2 tsp. toasted sesame oil
- 1 block firm tofu, sliced into cubes
- 1 tbsp. potato starch
- Cooking spray

Direction

1. In a bowl, mix the vinegar, soy sauce, and sesame oil.
2. Marinate the tofu for 30 minutes.
3. Coat the tofu with potato starch.
4. Spray the Ninja Foodi basket with oil.
5. Seal the crisping lid.
6. Choose the air crisp setting.
7. Cook at 370 degrees for 20 minutes, flipping halfway through.
8. You can serve with soy sauce and vinegar dipping sauce. Enjoy!

Onion Rings

Servings: 4

Total Time: 40 Minutes

Calories: 147

Fat: 11.3 g

Protein: 2.6 g

Carbs: 10.9 g

Ingredients and Quantity

- 3 yellow onions, sliced into rings
- 1/2 cup almond flour
- 2/3 cup unsweetened coconut milk
- 1/2 tsp. paprika
- 1/4 tsp. turmeric
- Salt, to taste

Direction

1. Mix all the ingredients except the onion rings in a large bowl.
2. Coat each onion ring with the mixture.
3. Place in the Ninja Foodi basket.
4. Seal the crisping lid.
5. Set it to air crisp.
6. Cook at 400 degrees for 10 minutes, flipping halfway through.
7. You can serve with ketchup or hot sauce. Enjoy!

Potato Wedges

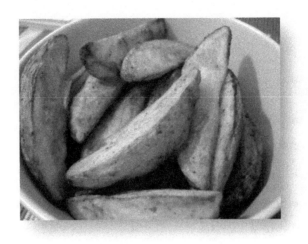

Servings: 4

Total Time: 40 Minutes

Calories: 179

Fat: 2.6 g

Protein: 2.8 g

Carbs: 36.2 g

Ingredients and Quantity

- 1 lb. potatoes, sliced into wedges
- 1 tsp. olive oil

- Salt and pepper, to taste
- 1/2 tsp. garlic powder

Direction

1. Coat the potatoes with oil.
2. Season with salt, pepper and garlic powder
3. Add the potatoes in the Ninja Foodi basket.
4. Cover with the crisping lid.
5. Set it to air crisp.
6. Cook at 400 degrees F for 16 minutes, flipping halfway through.
7. You can serve with vegan cheese sauce. Enjoy!

Garlic Chips

Servings: 2

Total Time: 70 Minutes

Calories: 156

Fat: 0.2 g

Protein: 4 g

Carbs: 35.4 g

Ingredients and Quantity

- Potatoes, sliced into chips
- Salt, to taste
- 4 garlic cloves
- 4 garlic cloves, minced
- 2 tbsp. vegan cheese

Direction

1. Put the potatoes in a bowl of water
2. Stir in the salt.
3. Soak for 20 to 30 minutes.
4. Drain the potatoes and pat try.
5. Season with the garlic and vegan cheese.
6. Arrange the chips on the Ninja Foodi basket.
7. Seal the crisping lid.
8. Set it to air crisp function.
9. Cook at 350 degrees for 10 minutes or until crispy.
10. Flip every 3 to 5 minutes.
11. You can serve with hot sauce or mayo. Enjoy!

Cauliflower Stir Fry

Servings: 4

Total Time: 40 Minutes

Calories: 93

Fat: 3 g

Protein: 4 g

Carbs: 12 g

Ingredients and Quantity

- 1 head cauliflower, sliced into florets
- 3/4 cup white onion, sliced
- 5 garlic cloves, minced
- 1 1/2 tsp. tamari
- 1 tbsp. rice vinegar
- 1/2 tsp. coconut sugar
- 1 tbsp. coconut cream

Direction

1. Put the cauliflower in the Ninja Foodi basket.
2. Seal the crisping lid.
3. Select the air crisp setting.
4. Cook at 350 degrees F for 10 minutes.
5. Add the onion, stir and cook for additional 10 minutes.
6. Add the garlic, and cook for 5 minutes.
7. Mix the rest of the ingredients.
8. Pour over the cauliflower before serving.
9. You can garnish with chopped scallions. Enjoy!

Vegan Cheese Sticks

Servings: 3

Total Time: 8 Hours 40 Minutes

Calories: 116

Fat: 4.1 g

Protein: 12.7 g

Carbs: 9.7 g

Ingredients and Quantity

- 1 block vegan mozzarella, sliced into strips
- 1 bag vegan chips
- 1 1/2 cups almond flour
- 2 cups coconut milk
- 1/4 cup nutritional yeast

Direction

1. Put the chips and nutritional yeast in the food processor.
2. Pulse until powdery.

3. Dip each cheese strip in the milk and cover with flour.

4. Dip into the milk again and coat with the powdered chips.

5. Place in the freezer for 8 hours.

6. Add the frozen cheese sticks to the Ninja Foodi basket.

7. Seal the crisping lid.

8. Set it to air crisp.

9. Cook at 380 degrees for 10 minutes.

10. You can serve with vegetable sticks. Enjoy!

Smoked Chickpeas

Servings: 3

Total Time: 45 Minutes

Calories: 423

Fat: 10.1 g

Protein: 20.8 g

Carbs: 65.2 g

Ingredients and Quantity

- 15 oz. chickpeas, rinsed and drained
- 1 tbsp. sunflower oil
- 2 tbsp. smoked paprika
- 1/2 tsp. granulated garlic
- 1/2 tsp. ground cumin
- 1/4 tsp. granulated onion
- Salt, to taste

Direction

1. Mix all the ingredients except the oil and chickpeas.
2. Put the chickpeas in the Ninja Foodi basket.
3. Seal the crisping lid.
4. Set it to air crisp function.
5. Cook at 390 degrees F for 15 minutes, shaking halfway through.
6. Put the chickpeas in the bowl of seasonings.
7. Put them back to the Ninja Foodi basket.
8. Cook at 360 degrees F for 3 minutes.
9. You can add cayenne pepper to make the dish spicier. Enjoy!

Fried Broccoli

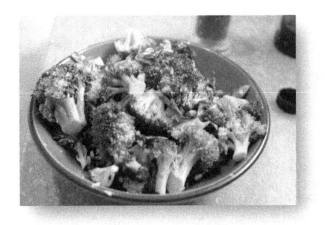

Servings: 2

Total Time: 25 Minutes

Calories: 197

Fat: 14.5 g

Protein: 7.4 g

Carbs: 14.4 g

Ingredients and Quantity

- 4 cups broccoli florets
- 2 tbsp. coconut oil

- 1 tbsp. nutritional yeast
- Salt and pepper, to taste

Direction

1. Combine all the ingredients in a bowl.
2. Place the broccoli in the Ninja Foodi basket.
3. Seal the crisping lid.
4. Choose air crisp setting.
5. Cook at 370 degrees F for 5 minutes.
6. You can serve as side dish. Enjoy!

Garlic Pepper Potato Chips

Servings: 2

Total Time: 30 Minutes

Calories: 197

Fat: 14.5 g

Protein: 7.4 g

Carbs: 14.4 g

Ingredients and Quantity

- 1 large potato, sliced into thin chips
- Cooking spray
- Salt and garlic powder, to taste
- 1 tsp. black pepper

Direction

1. Spray oil on the Ninja Foodi basket.
2. Season the potato with the salt, garlic powder and black pepper.

3. Place potato chips on the basket.

4. Seal the crisping lid.

5. Set it to air crisp.

6. Cook at 450 degrees F for 10 minutes or until golden and crispy.

7. You can serve with mayo dip. Enjoy!

Crispy Brussels Sprouts

Servings: 4

Total Time: 30 Minutes

Calories: 139

Fat: 5.4 g

Protein: 7.8 g

Carbs: 20.9 g

Ingredients and Quantity

- 1 lb. Brussels sprouts
- 2 tbsp. olive oil
- 1/4 tsp. garlic powder
- 1/4 tsp. salt

Direction

1. Put the Brussels sprouts in a bowl.
2. Pour the olive oil into the bowl.
3. Season the sprouts with garlic powder and salt.

4. Put the sprouts on the basket.
5. Seal the crisping lid.
6. Set it to air crisp function.
7. Cook at 370 degrees F for 6 minutes, flipping halfway through.
8. 8. You can serve as side dish. Enjoy!

Veggie Fritters

Servings: 6

Total Time: 45 Minutes

Calories: 171

Fat: 0.5 g

Protein: 5.8 g

Carbs: 35.7 g

Ingredients and Quantity

- 3 tbsp. ground flaxseed mixed with 1/2 cup water
- 2 potatoes, shredded
- 2 cups frozen mixed veggies
- 1 cup frozen peas, thawed
- 1/2 cup onion, chopped
- 1/4 cup fresh cilantro, chopped
- 1/2 cup almond flour
- Salt, to taste
- Cooking spray

Direction

1. Combine all the ingredients in a bowl and then form patties.
2. Spray each patty with oil.
3. Transfer to the Ninja Foodi basket.
4. Set it to air crisp.
5. Close the crisping lid.
6. Cook at 360 degrees F for 15 minutes, flipping halfway through.
7. Transfer to a serving plate. Serve and enjoy!

Steamed Broccoli and Carrots with Lemon

Servings: 3

Total Time: 10 Minutes

Calories: 35

Fat: 0.3 g

Protein: 1.7 g

Carbs: 8.1 g

Ingredients and Quantity

- 1 cup broccoli florets
- 1/2 cup carrots, julienned
- 2 tbsp. lemon juice
- Salt and pepper, to taste

Direction

1. Place the Ninja Foodi Cook and Crisp reversible rack inside the ceramic pot.
2. Pour water into the pot.
3. Toss everything in a mixing bowl and combine.
4. Place the vegetables on the reversible rack.
5. Close the pressure lid and set the vent to SEAL.
6. Press the Steam button and adjust the cooking time to 10 minutes.
7. Do a quick pressure, release. Serve and enjoy!

Crusty Sweet Potato Hash

Servings: 4

Total Time: 15 Minutes

Calories: 195

Fat: 6 g

Protein: 3.7 g

Carbs: 31.4 g

Ingredients and Quantity

- 2 large sweet potatoes, cut into small cubes
- slices bacon, cut into small pieces
- 2 tbsp. olive oil
- 1 tbsp. smoked paprika
- 2 tsp. salt
- 1 tsp. ground black pepper
- tsp. dill weed

Direction

1. Place in the ceramic pot the Ninja Foodi Cook and Crisp basket.
2. Combine all ingredients in a bowl and give a good stir.
3. Form small patties using your hands.
4. Place the patties in the basket.
5. Close the crisping lid and press the Air Crisp button before pressing the START button.
6. Adjust the cooking time to 10 minutes.
7. Flip the patties halfway through the cooking time for even cooking. Serve and enjoy!

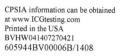

CPSIA information can be obtained
at www.ICGtesting.com
Printed in the USA
BVHW041407270421
605944BV00006B/1408